Plant Based

Diet Cookbook for Beginners

Budget-Friendly Recipes for Plant-Based Eating All Through the Year

Jacqueline Bachman

TABLE OF CONTENTS

INTRODUCTION

A plant-based diet is a diet that promotes eating all, or almost all, foods that come from plants. In practice, this usually means eating only plant-based foods, but some people may occasionally eat animal products as well. eating a plant based diet is the best way to get your protein. You should eat meat sparingly because it's hard for the body to break down. Eating meat is linked to cancer, heart disease, and early death.

A plant-based diet is a diet that focuses on the consumption of plant-based foods. Plants based food are the foundation of a healthy diet, and they offer a wide variety of vitamins, minerals, fiber, and antioxidants that often are missing from other diets. Plant based diets are usually vegan diets, but they can also be vegetarian diets. A vegan diet refers to that you don't eat any animal products, including meat, dairy, and eggs. A vegetarian diet on the other means that you don't eat meat, but you might eat dairy and eggs.

It is not difficult to prepare delicious meals using only plant-based whole foods. It's best to be creative if you want to get the most nutrients out of your diet. Start with whole grain breads, whole grain pasta, steel cut oats, colorful fruits, and raw vegetables as a foundation. Then you would be more inventive:

Toss your oatmeal with fruits and spices.

Flax seed can be added to your whole grain cereal.

Make salad the main course for lunch or dinner, and be inventive with it.

Vegetables of your preference can be added to whole grain pasta or rice.

Blend as many fruits and vegetables as possible into smoothies.

Toss whole grain bread with plant-based, natural nut butters.

Dessert should consist of berries.

Beans may be added to lunch and dinner entrees.

Every meal should include at least one fruit or vegetable.

BREAKFAST RECIPES

1. Tropi-Kale Breeze

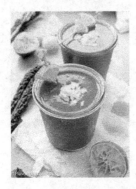

Preparation time: 5 minutes

Cooking time: 0 minutes

Servings: 3-4

Ingredients:

- 1 cup chopped pineapple (frozen or fresh)

- 1 cup chopped mango (frozen or fresh)

- ½ to 1 cup chopped kale

- ½ avocado

- ½ cup of coconut milk

- 1 cup water or coconut water

- 1 teaspoon matcha green tea powder (optional)

Directions:

1. Purée everything in a blender until smooth, adding more water (or coconut milk) if needed.

Nutrition: Calories: 566 Fat: 36g Carbs: 66g Protein: 8g

2. Hydration Station

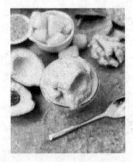

Preparation time: 5 minutes

Cooking time: 0 minutes

Servings: 3-4

Ingredients:

- 1 banana
- 1 orange, peeled and sectioned, or 1 cup pure orange juice
- 1 cup strawberries (frozen or fresh)
- 1 cup chopped cucumber
- ½ cup of coconut water
- 1 cup of water
- ½ cup ice

Bonus boosters (optional):

- 1 cup chopped spinach
- ¼ cup fresh mint, chopped

Directions:

1. Purée everything in a blender until smooth, adding more water if needed. Add bonus boosters, as desired. Purée until blended.

Nutrition: Calories: 320 Fat: 3g Carbs: 76g Protein: 6g

3. Mango Madness

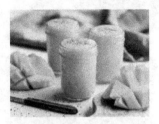

Preparation time: 5 minutes

Cooking time: 0 minutes

Servings: 3-4

Ingredients:

- 1 banana
- 1 cup chopped mango (frozen or fresh)
- 1 cup chopped peach (frozen or fresh)
- 1 cup strawberries
- 1 carrot, peeled and chopped (optional)
- 1 cup of water

Directions:

1. Purée everything in a blender until smooth, adding more water if needed.

Nutrition: Calories: 376 Fat: 2g Carbs: 95g Protein: 5g

4. Chocolate PB Smoothie

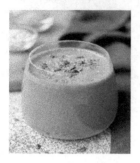

Preparation time: 5 minutes

Cooking time: 0 minutes

Servings: 3-4

Ingredients:

- 1 banana
- ¼ cup rolled oats or 1 scoop plant protein powder
- 1 tablespoon flaxseed or chia seeds
- 1 tablespoon unsweetened cocoa powder
- 1 tablespoon peanut butter, or almond or sunflower seed butter
- 1 tablespoon maple syrup (optional)
- 1 cup alfalfa sprouts or spinach, chopped (optional)
- ½ cup non-dairy milk (optional)
- 1 cup of water

Bonus boosters (optional):

- 1 teaspoon maca powder
- 1 teaspoon cocoa nibs

Directions:

1. Purée everything in a blender until smooth, adding more water (or non-dairy milk) if needed. Add bonus boosters, as desired. Purée until blended.

Nutrition: Calories: 474 Fat: 16g Carbs: 79g Protein: 13g

5. Pink Panther Smoothie

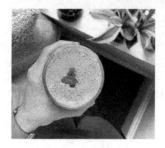

Preparation time: 5 minutes

Cooking time: 0 minutes

Servings: 3

Ingredients:

- 1 cup strawberries
- 1 cup chopped melon (any kind)
- 1 cup cranberries or raspberries
- 1 tablespoon chia seeds
- ½ cup coconut milk, or other non-dairy milk
- 1 cup of water

Bonus boosters (optional):

- 1 teaspoon goji berries
- 2 tablespoons fresh mint, chopped

Directions:

1. Purée everything in a blender until smooth, adding more water (or coconut milk) if needed. Add bonus boosters, as desired. Purée until blended.

Nutrition: Calories: 459 Fat: 30g Carbs: 52g Protein: 8g

6. Banana Nut Smoothie

Preparation time: 5 minutes

Cooking time: 0 minutes

Servings: 2-3

Ingredients:

- 1 banana
- 1 tablespoon almond butter/sunflower seed butter
- ¼ teaspoon ground cinnamon
- Pinch ground nutmeg
- 1 to 2 tablespoons dates or maple syrup
- 1 tablespoon ground flaxseed, or chia, or hemp hearts
- ½ cup non-dairy milk (optional)
- 1 cup of water

Directions:

1. Purée everything in a blender until smooth, adding more water (or non-dairy milk) if needed.

Nutrition: Calories: 343 Fat: 14g Carbs: 55g Protein: 6g

7. Oatmeal Breakfast Cookies

Preparation time: 15 minutes

Cooking time: 12 minutes

Servings: 5

Ingredients:

- 1 tablespoon ground flaxseed
- 2 tablespoons almond butter/sunflower seed butter
- 2 tablespoons maple syrup
- 1 banana, mashed
- 1 teaspoon ground cinnamon
- ¼ teaspoon ground nutmeg (optional)
- Pinch sea salt
- ½ cup rolled oats
- ¼ cup raisins, or dark chocolate chips

Directions:

1. Preheat the oven to 350°F. Prepare your large baking sheet lined with parchment paper. Mix the ground flax with just enough water to cover it in a small dish, and leave it to sit.

2. In a large bowl, mix the almond butter and maple syrup until creamy, then add the banana. Add the flax-water mixture.

3. Sift the cinnamon, nutmeg, and salt into a separate medium bowl, then stir into the wet mixture. Add the oats and raisins, and fold in.

4. Form 3 to 4 tablespoons batter into a ball and press lightly to flatten onto the baking sheet. Repeat, spacing the cookies 2 to 3 inches apart.

5. Bake within 12 minutes, or until golden brown. Store the cookies in an airtight container in the fridge, or freeze them for later.

Nutrition: Calories: 192 Fat: 6g Carbs: 34g Protein: 4g

8. Sunshine Muffins

Preparation time: 15 minutes

Cooking time: 30 minutes

Servings: 6

Ingredients:

- 1 teaspoon coconut oil for greasing muffin tins (optional)
- 2 tablespoons almond butter/sunflower seed butter
- ¼ cup non-dairy milk
- 1 orange, peeled
- 1 carrot, coarsely chopped
- 2 tablespoons chopped dried apricots/other dried fruit
- 3 tablespoons molasses
- 2 tablespoons ground flaxseed
- 1 teaspoon apple cider vinegar
- 1 teaspoon pure vanilla extract
- ½ teaspoon ground cinnamon
- ½ teaspoon ground ginger (optional)
- ¼ teaspoon ground nutmeg (optional)
- ¼ teaspoon allspice (optional)
- ¾ cup rolled oats or whole-grain flour

- 1 teaspoon baking powder
- ½ teaspoon baking soda

Mix-ins (optional):

- ½ cup rolled oats
- 2 tablespoons raisins or other chopped dried fruit
- 2 tablespoons sunflower seeds

Directions:

1. Preheat the oven to 350°F. Prepare a 6-cup muffin tin by rubbing the cups' insides with coconut oil or using silicone or paper muffin cups.

2. Purée the nut butter, milk, orange, carrot, apricots, molasses, flaxseed, vinegar, vanilla, cinnamon, ginger, nutmeg, and allspice in a food processor or blender until somewhat smooth.

3. Grind the oats in a clean coffee grinder until they're consistent with flour (or use whole-grain flour). In a large bowl, mix the oats with the baking powder and baking soda.

4. Mix the wet ingredients into the dry ingredients until just combined. Fold in the mix-ins (if using).

5. Spoon about ¼ cup batter into each muffin cup and bake for 30 minutes, or until a toothpick inserted into the center comes out clean.

Nutrition: Calories: 287 Fat: 12g Carbs: 41g Protein: 8g

9. Applesauce Crumble Muffins

Preparation time: 15 minutes

Cooking time: 15-20 minutes

Servings: 12

Ingredients:

- 1 teaspoon coconut oil for greasing muffin tins (optional)
- 2 tablespoons nut butter or seed butter
- 1½ cups unsweetened applesauce
- 1/3 cup coconut sugar
- ½ cup non-dairy milk
- 2 tablespoons ground flaxseed
- 1 teaspoon apple cider vinegar
- 1 teaspoon pure vanilla extract
- 2 cups whole-grain flour
- 1 teaspoon baking soda
- ½ teaspoon baking powder
- 1 teaspoon ground cinnamon
- Pinch sea salt
- ½ cup walnuts, chopped

Toppings (optional):

- ¼ cup walnuts
- ¼ cup of coconut sugar
- ½ teaspoon ground cinnamon

Directions:

1. Preheat the oven to 350°F. Prepare two 6-cup muffin tins by rubbing the cups' insides with coconut oil or using silicone or paper muffin cups.
2. In a large bowl, mix the nut butter, applesauce, coconut sugar, milk, flaxseed, vinegar, and vanilla until thoroughly combined, or purée in a food processor or blender.
3. In another large bowl, sift together the flour, baking soda, baking powder, cinnamon, salt, and chopped walnuts. Mix the dry ingredients into the wet ingredients until just combined.
4. Spoon about ¼ cup batter into each muffin cup and sprinkle with the topping of your choice (if using). Bake for 15 to 20 minutes, or until a toothpick inserted into the center comes out clean.

Nutrition: Calories: 287 Fat: 12g Carbs: 41g Protein: 8g

10. Baked Banana French Toast with Raspberry Syrup

Preparation time: 10 minutes

Cooking time: 30 minutes

Servings: 8 slices

Ingredients:

For the French toast:

- 1 banana
- 1 cup of coconut milk
- 1 teaspoon pure vanilla extract
- ¼ teaspoon ground nutmeg
- ½ teaspoon ground cinnamon
- 1½ teaspoons arrowroot powder or flour
- Pinch sea salt
- 8 slices whole-grain bread

For the raspberry syrup:

- 1 cup raspberries/other berries
- 2 tablespoons water, or pure fruit juice
- 1 to 2 tablespoons maple syrup or coconut sugar (optional)

Directions:

1. For the French toast, preheat the oven to 350°F. In a shallow bowl, purée or mash the banana well. Mix in the coconut milk, vanilla, nutmeg, cinnamon, arrowroot, and salt.

2. Dip the slices of bread in the banana mixture, and then lay them out in a 13-by-9-inch baking dish. They should cover the bottom of the dish and overlap slightly but shouldn't be stacked on top of each other.

3. Pour any leftover banana mixture over the bread, and put the dish in the oven—Bake within 30 minutes, or until the tops are lightly browned. Serve topped with raspberry syrup.

To Make the Raspberry Syrup:

1. Heat the raspberries in a small pot with the water and the maple syrup (if using) on medium heat.

2. Leave to simmer, stirring occasionally, and breaking up the berries for 15 to 20 minutes, until the liquid has reduced.

Nutrition: Calories: 166 Fat: 7g Carbs: 23g Protein: 5g

LUNCH

11. Chickpea and Avocado Salad

Preparation time: 5 minutes

Cooking time: 0 minutes

Servings: 4

Ingredients:

- 1 ½ cup cooked chickpeas
- 1 medium avocado
- ¼ teaspoon salt
- ¼ teaspoon ground black pepper
- ¼ cup chopped cilantro
- 2 tablespoons chopped green onion
- 3 tablespoons lime juice

Directions:

1. Place chickpeas in a medium bowl and then mash with a fork.
2. Add avocado into the chickpeas, mash with a fork, add green onion and cilantro, drizzle with lime juice, and season with salt and black pepper.

3. Serve the chickpea salad on bread as a sandwich.

Nutrition: Calories: 234 Fat: 8 g Protein: 10 g Carbs: 33 g

12. Spinach and Orange Salad

Preparation time: 5 minutes

Cooking time: 0 minutes

Servings: 6

Ingredients:

- 10 ounces fresh spinach
- 1 teaspoon Brazil nuts
- 10 strawberries, sliced
- 1 teaspoon sunflower seeds
- 10 ounces canned clementine oranges
- ¼ cup raspberry vinaigrette

Directions:

1. Take a medium bowl, place all the ingredients in it and then toss until coated. Serve straight away.

Nutrition: Calories: 109 Fat: 2 g Protein: 3 g Carbs: 18 g

13. **Pesto Broccoli Rice**

Preparation time: 5 minutes

Cooking time: 8 minutes

Servings: 6

Ingredients:

- 4 cups of broccoli rice
- ¼ teaspoon salt
- ¼ teaspoon ground black pepper
- ¾ cup kale pesto
- 1 tablespoon olive oil
- 4 tablespoons grated parmesan cheese, vegan
- 1 lemon, cut into wedges

Directions:

1. Put your large saucepan on medium heat, add oil, and let it heat. Add broccoli rice, stir until mixed, and then cook for 4 minutes until tender.

2. Remove pan from heat, add pesto, stir until mixed, and then remove the pan from heat. Season with salt and black pepper, add parmesan cheese, and then distribute broccoli rice among four bowls. Serve broccoli rice with a lime wedge.

Nutrition: Calories: 42 Fat: 3 g Protein: 2 g Carbs: 4 g

14. **Roasted Tomatoes**

Preparation time: 5 minutes

Cooking time: 25 minutes

Servings: 3

Ingredients:

- 3 ½ cups halved cherry tomatoes
- 3 teaspoons minced garlic
- ½ teaspoon salt
- 1 tablespoon minced basil
- ¼ teaspoon red chili flakes
- ½ teaspoon balsamic vinegar
- 1 tablespoon olive oil
- 1 tablespoon minced parsley

Directions:

1. Switch on the oven, then set it to 375 degrees F and let it preheat. Take a large bowl, place all the ingredients in it and then toss until mixed.

2. Take a baking sheet, line it with a parchment sheet, spread tomato mixture, and then bake for 25 minutes until roasted. Serve straight away.

Nutrition: Calories: 115.6 Fat: 9.6 g Protein: 1.6 g Carbs: 8 g

15. Asparagus Soup

Preparation time: 5 minutes

Cooking time: 28 minutes

Servings: 6

Ingredients:

- 4 pounds potatoes, peeled, chopped
- 1 bunch of asparagus
- 15 ounces cooked cannellini beans
- 1 small white onion, peeled, diced
- 3 teaspoons minced garlic
- 1 teaspoon grated ginger
- ½ teaspoon salt
- ¼ teaspoon ground black pepper
- 1 lemon, juiced
- 1 tablespoon olive oil
- 8 cups vegetable broth

Directions:

1. Place oil in a large pot, place it over medium heat, and heat until hot. Add onion into the pot, stir in garlic and ginger and then cook for 5 minutes until onion turns tender.

2. Add potatoes, asparagus, and beans, pour in the broth, stir until mixed, and then bring the mixture to a boil.

3. Cook the potatoes for 20 minutes until tender, remove the pot from heat, and then puree half of the soup until smooth.

4. Add salt, black pepper, and lemon juice, stir until mixed, ladle soup into bowls and then serve.

Nutrition: Calories: 123.3 Fat: 4.4 g Protein: 4.7 g Carbs: 16.3 g

16. Tofu and Pesto Sandwich

Preparation time: 5 minutes

Cooking time: 15 minutes

Servings: 4

Ingredients:

- 12 ounces of tofu, pressed, drained
- 4 leaves of butter lettuce
- 4 slices of tomato
- 4 tablespoons basil pesto
- 1 tablespoon olive oil
- 4 slices of whole-wheat sandwich bread

Directions:

1. Switch on the oven, then set it to 375 degrees F and let it preheat. Cut tofu into slices, place them in a bowl, drizzle with oil and then sprinkle with oregano.

2. Spread tofu pieces on a baking sheet and then roast for 15 minutes.

3. Assemble the sandwich and for this, spread 1 tablespoon of basil pesto on one side of each sandwich slice, top with a lettuce leaf, tomato slice, and tofu. Serve straight away.

Nutrition: Calories: 219 Fat: 13.5 g Protein: 8 g Carbs: 18.5 g

17. **Roasted Brussel Sprouts**

Preparation time: 5 minutes

Cooking time: 30 minutes

Servings: 4

Ingredients:

- 3 cups Brussel sprouts
- ½ cup dried cranberries
- 1 ½ teaspoon salt
- 1 teaspoon ground black pepper
- 2 tablespoons olive oil

Directions:

1. Switch on the oven, then set it to 375 degrees F and let it preheat. Meanwhile, cut each Brussel sprout in half and then place them in a large bowl.

2. Add salt and black pepper, drizzle with oil, toss until coated, and then spread on a baking sheet.

3. Add cranberries to it, and then roast the Brussel sprouts for 30 minutes until cooked. Serve straight away.

Nutrition: Calories: 135 Fat: 9.8 g Protein: 3.9 g Carbs: 11 g

18. <u>Vegetable with Brown Rice</u>

Preparation time: 5 minutes

Cooking time: 55 minutes

Servings: 4

Ingredients:

- 16-ounce extra-firm tofu, pressed, drained
- 1 cup broccoli florets
- 1 cup brown rice, rinsed
- 1 small white onion, peeled, diced
- 1 ½ tablespoon minced garlic
- 1 medium red bell pepper, cored, diced
- 1 tablespoon olive oil
- 2 cups of water

Directions:

1. Take a medium pot, place it over medium-high heat, add rice, pour in the water, and then bring to a boil.

2. Then switch heat to medium-low level, cover the pot with the lid and then cook the rice for 40 minutes, set aside until required. Place oil in a large skillet pan, place it over medium-high heat, and let it heat.

3. Cut tofu into ½-inch cubes, add into the pan and broccoli, onion, bell pepper, and garlic, and then cook for 5 minutes until vegetables become tender.

4. Add rice into the pan, toss until mixed, and then cook for 5 minutes until hot. Serve straight away.

Nutrition: Calories: 279.4 Fat: 8 g Protein: 10.5 g Carbs: 45.8 g

19. Tomato and Basil Spaghetti

Preparation time: 5 minutes

Cooking time: 10 minutes

Servings: 4

Ingredients:

- 1 pound angel hair spaghetti, cooked
- 15 ounces cooked northern beans
- 10 1/2 ounces cherry tomatoes, halved
- 1 small white onion, peeled, diced
- 8 basil leaves, chopped
- 1 ½ tablespoon minced garlic
- 2 tablespoons olive oil
- 1 cup of pasta water

Directions:

1. Take a large pot, place it over medium-high heat, and then cook pasta according to its package instructions, reserving 1 cup of pasta water.

2. Take a large skillet pan, place it over medium-high heat, add oil and let it heat until hot. Add onion, tomatoes, garlic, and basil, and then cook for 5 minutes until the vegetables turn tender.

3. Add pasta and beans, pour in the pasta water, and then toss until coated. Serve straight away.

Nutrition: Calories: 147 Fat: 5 g Protein: 3.8 g Carbs: 21.2 g

20. Pasta Salad

Preparation time: 10 minutes

Cooking time: 25 minutes

Servings: 4

Ingredients:

- 1 medium zucchini, sliced
- ½ cup cherry tomatoes
- ¼ cup frozen peas
- 1 teaspoon salt
- ½ teaspoon ground black pepper
- 1 teaspoon hemp seeds
- 3 cups fusilli pasta

Directions:

1. Switch on the oven, then set it to 375 degrees F and let it preheat. Spread the cherry tomatoes on a baking sheet and then bake for 15 minutes until roasted.

2. In the meantime, take a large pot, place it over medium-high heat, cook pasta according to the instructions on its package, and then drain it.

3. Meanwhile, take a griddle pan, place it over medium-high heat and then grease it with oil. Put the zucchini

slices on your pan and then cook for 3 minutes per side until golden brown.

4. Take a small pot, place it over medium-low heat, add peas, cover with water and then boil them for 10 minutes.

5. When done, drain the peas, rinse under cold water, and then set aside until required. Put the cooked pasta in your large bowl, add basil, salt, and black pepper and then toss until mixed.

6. Add remaining ingredients into the salad bowl, toss until combined, and then serve.

Nutrition: Calories: 144 Fat: 5.4 g Protein: 3.1 g Carbs: 21.2 g

DINNER

21. Dijon Maple Burgers

Preparation Time: 20 minutes

Cooking Time: 30 minutes

Servings: 12

Ingredients:

- 1 red bell pepper
- 19 ounces can chickpeas, rinsed & drained
- 1 cup almonds, ground
- 2 teaspoons Dijon mustard
- 1 teaspoon oregano
- ½ teaspoon sage
- 1 cup spinach, fresh
- 1 – ½ cups rolled oats
- 1 clove garlic, pressed
- ½ lemon, juiced
- 2 teaspoons maple syrup, pure

Directions:

1. Get out a baking sheet. Line it with parchment paper. Cut your red pepper in half and then take the seeds out. Place it on your baking sheet, and roast in the oven while you prepare your other ingredients.

2. Process your chickpeas, almonds, mustard, and maple syrup together in a food processor. Add in your lemon juice, oregano, sage, garlic, and spinach, processing again. Make sure it's combined, but don't puree it.

3. Once your red bell pepper is softened, which should roughly take ten minutes, add this to the processor as well. Add in your oats, mixing well.

4. Form twelve patties, cooking in the oven for a half-hour. They should be browned.

Nutrition: Calories: 96 Protein: 5.28 g Fat: 2.42 g Carbohydrates: 16.82 g

22. Black Lentil Curry

Preparation Time: 30 minutes

Cooking Time: 6 hours and 15 minutes

Servings: 4

Ingredients:

- 1 cup of black lentils, rinsed and soaked overnight
- 14 ounces of chopped tomatoes
- 2 large white onions, peeled and sliced
- 1 1/2 teaspoon of minced garlic
- 1 teaspoon of grated ginger
- 1 red chili
- 1 teaspoon of salt
- 1/4 teaspoon of red chili powder
- 1 teaspoon of paprika
- 1 teaspoon of ground turmeric
- 2 teaspoons of ground cumin
- 2 teaspoons of ground coriander
- 1/2 cup of chopped coriander
- 4-ounce of vegetarian butter
- 4 fluid of ounce water
- 2 fluid of ounce vegetarian double cream

Directions:

1. Place a large pan over moderate heat, add butter and let heat until melt. Add the onion and garlic and ginger and cook for 10 to 15 minutes or until onions are caramelized.

2. Then stir in salt, red chili powder, paprika, turmeric, cumin, ground coriander, and water. Transfer this mixture to a 6-quarts slow cooker and add tomatoes and red chili.

3. Drain lentils, add to slow cooker, and stir until just mix. Plugin slow cooker; adjust cooking time to 6 hours and let cook on low heat setting.

4. When the lentils are done, stir in cream and adjust the seasoning. Serve with boiled rice or whole wheat bread.

Nutrition: Calories: 299 Protein: 5.59 g Fat: 27.92 g Carbohydrates: 9.83 g

23. Flavorful Refried Beans

Preparation Time: 15 minutes

Cooking Time: 8 hours

Servings: 8

Ingredients:

- 3 cups of pinto beans, rinsed
- 1 small jalapeno pepper, seeded and chopped
- 1 medium-sized white onion, peeled and sliced
- 2 tablespoons of minced garlic
- 5 teaspoons of salt
- 2 teaspoons of ground black pepper
- 1/4 teaspoon of ground cumin
- 9 cups of water

Directions:

1. Using a 6-quarts slow cooker, place all the ingredients and stir until it mixes properly. Cover the top, plug in the slow cooker, adjust the cooking time to 6 hours, let it cook on the high heat setting, and add more water if the beans get too dry.

2. When the beans are done, drain it then reserve the liquid. Mash the beans using a potato masher and pour

in the reserved cooking liquid until it reaches your desired mixture. Serve immediately.

Nutrition: Calories: 268 Protein: 16.55 g Fat: 1.7 g Carbohydrates: 46.68 g

24. Smoky Red Beans and Rice

Preparation Time: 15 minutes

Cooking Time: 6 minutes

Servings: 6

Ingredients:

- 30 ounces of cooked red beans
- 1 cup of brown rice, uncooked
- 1 cup of chopped green pepper
- 1 cup of chopped celery
- 1 cup of chopped white onion
- 1 1/2 teaspoon of minced garlic
- 1/2 teaspoon of salt
- 1/4 teaspoon of cayenne pepper
- 1 teaspoon of smoked paprika
- 2 teaspoons of dried thyme
- 1 bay leaf
- 2 1/3 cups of vegetable broth

Directions:

1. Using a 6-quarts slow cooker, place all the ingredients except for the rice, salt, and cayenne pepper. Stir until it mixes properly and then cover the top.

2. Plug in the slow cooker, adjust the cooking time to 4 hours, and steam on a low heat setting.

3. Then pour in and stir the rice, salt, cayenne pepper and continue cooking for an additional 2 hours at a high heat setting. Serve straight away.

Nutrition: Calories: 791 Protein: 3.25 g Fat: 86.45 g Carbohydrates: 9.67 g

25. Spicy Black-Eyed Peas

Preparation Time: 12 minutes

Cooking Time: 8 hours and 8 minutes

Servings: 8

Ingredients:

- 32-ounce black-eyed peas, uncooked
- 1 cup of chopped orange bell pepper
- 1 cup of chopped celery
- 8-ounce of chipotle peppers, chopped
- 1 cup of chopped carrot
- 1 cup of chopped white onion
- 1 teaspoon of minced garlic
- 3/4 teaspoon of salt
- 1/2 teaspoon of ground black pepper
- 2 teaspoons of liquid smoke flavoring
- 2 teaspoons of ground cumin
- 1 tablespoon of adobo sauce
- 2 tablespoons of olive oil
- 1 tablespoon of apple cider vinegar
- 4 cups of vegetable broth

Directions:

1. Place a medium-sized non-stick skillet pan over an average temperature of heat; add the bell peppers, carrot, onion, garlic, oil, and vinegar.

2. Stir until it mixes properly and let it cook for 5 to 8 minutes or until it gets translucent.

3. Transfer this mixture to a 6-quarts slow cooker and add the peas, chipotle pepper, adobo sauce, and the vegetable broth. Stir until mixed properly and cover the top.

4. Plug in the slow cooker, adjust the cooking time to 8 hours, and let it cook on the low heat setting or until peas are soft. Serve right away.

Nutrition: Calories: 1071 Protein: 5.3 g Fat: 113.65 g Carbohydrates: 18.51 g

26. Creamy Artichoke Soup

Preparation Time: 5 minutes

Cooking Time: 40 minutes

Servings: 4

Ingredients:

- 1 can artichoke hearts, drained
- 3 cups vegetable broth
- 2 tbsp. lemon juice
- 1 small onion, finely cut
- 2 cloves garlic, crushed
- 3 tbsp. olive oil
- 2 tbsp. flour
- ½ cup vegan cream

Directions:

1. Gently sauté the onion and garlic in some olive oil. Add the flour, whisking constantly, and then add the hot vegetable broth slowly, while still whisking. Cook for about 5 minutes.

2. Blend the artichoke, lemon juice, salt, and pepper until smooth. Add the puree to the broth mix, stir well, and then stir in the cream.

3. Cook until heated through. Garnish with a swirl of vegan cream or a sliver of artichoke.

Nutrition: Calories: 1622 Protein: 4.45 g Fat: 181.08 g Carbohydrates: 10.99 g

27. Tomato Artichoke Soup

Preparation Time: 5 minutes

Cooking Time: 35 minutes

Servings: 4

Ingredients:

- 1 can artichoke hearts, drained
- 1 can diced tomatoes, undrained
- 3 cups vegetable broth
- 1 small onion, chopped
- 2 cloves garlic, crushed
- 1 tbsp. pesto
- Black pepper, to taste

Directions:

1. Combine all ingredients in the slow cooker. Cover and cook on low within 8-10 hours or on high within 4-5 hours.
2. Blend the soup in batches then put it back to the slow cooker. Season with pepper and salt, then serve.

Nutrition: Calories: 1487 Protein: 3.98 g Fat: 167.42 g Carbohydrates: 8.2 g

28. <u>Super Radish Avocado Salad</u>

Preparation Time: 10 minutes

Cooking Time: 0 minutes

Servings: 2

Ingredients:

- 6 shredded carrots
- 6 ounces diced radishes
- 1 diced avocado
- 1/3 cup ponzu

Directions:

1. Place all together the ingredients in a serving bowl and toss. Enjoy!

Nutrition: Calories: 292 Protein: 7.42 g Fat: 18.29 g Carbohydrates: 29.59 g

29. Beauty School Ginger Cucumbers

Preparation Time: 10 minutes

Cooking Time: 0 minutes

Servings: 2

Ingredients:

- 1 sliced cucumber
- 3 tsp. rice wine vinegar
- 1 ½ tbsp. sugar
- 1 tsp. minced ginger

Directions:

1. Place all together the ingredients in a mixing bowl, and toss the ingredients well. Enjoy!

Nutrition: Calories: 10 Protein: 0.46 g Fat: 0.43 g Carbohydrates: 0.89 g

30. <u>Butternut Squash and Chickpea Curry</u>

Preparation Time: 20 minutes

Cooking Time: 6 hours

Servings: 8

Ingredients:

- 1 1/2 cups of shelled peas
- 1 1/2 cups of chickpeas, uncooked and rinsed
- 2 1/2 cups of diced butternut squash
- 12 ounces of chopped spinach
- 2 large tomatoes, diced
- 1 small white onion, peeled and chopped
- 1 teaspoon of minced garlic
- 1 teaspoon of salt
- 3 tablespoons of curry powder
- 14-ounce of coconut milk
- 3 cups of vegetable broth
- 1/4 cup of chopped cilantro

Directions:

1. Using a 6-quarts slow cooker, place all the ingredients into it except for the spinach and peas.

2. Cover the top, plug in the slow cooker; adjust the cooking time to 6 hours, and cook on the high heat setting or until the chickpeas get tender.

3. 30 minutes to ending your cooking, add the peas and spinach to the slow cooker and cook for the remaining 30 minutes.

4. Stir to check the sauce; if the sauce is runny, stir in a mixture of a 1 tbsp. Cornstarch mixed with 2 tbsp water. Serve with boiled rice.

Nutrition: Calories: 774 Protein: 3.71 g Fat: 83.25 g Carbohydrates: 12.64 g

SNACKS

31. Fresh Edamame Pods with Aleppo Pepper

Preparation Time: 0 minutes

Cooking Time: 5 minutes

Servings: 1

Ingredients

- ½ cup Edamame (in pods)
- 1/8 tsp Aleppo pepper

Directions:

1. Start by taking a steamer and place it over high flame. Fill it with water and let it come to a boil.

2. Place the edamame pods in the steamer and steam for about 5 minutes. The pods should be crisp and tender. Transfer into a serving platter and sprinkle with Aleppo pepper.

Nutrition: Calories: 124 Carbs: 12g Fat: 4g Protein: 10g

32. Toast with Cannellini Beans and Pesto

Preparation Time: 5 minutes

Cooking Time: 0 minutes

Servings: 1

Ingredients:

- 1 slice Whole-wheat bread (toasted)
- 1/3 cup Canned cannellini beans (no-salt added)
- 1 pinch Garlic powder
- ½ teaspoon Basil pesto
- 2 tablespoons Tomato (chopped)

Directions:

1. Start by rinsing and draining the canned cannellini beans. Keep aside. Take the toasted slice and place it on a plate.

2. Take a small mixing bowl and add in the beans, tomatoes and garlic powder. Mix well. Place the prepared beans and tomatoes mixture on the toast and top with pesto. Serve.

Nutrition: Calories: 366 Carbs: 49g Fat: 12g Protein: 21g

33. <u>Popped Amaranth</u>

Preparation time: 15 minutes

Cooking time: 10-15 minutes

Servings: 2-3

Ingredients:

- ¼ cup whole amaranth
- 2 teaspoons refined coconut, sunflower, or avocado oil
- Sea salt

Directions:

1. Put your pan to just the right temperature. Place it over medium-high heat and add about 3 amaranth grains to the pot. Cover with the lid and watch.
2. Once the amaranth grains turn dark brown, discard and add just enough new amaranth to barely cover the bottom of the pot in a single layer.
3. As soon as those amaranth grains go in, immediately begin shaking the pot. The grains will begin to pop— don't stop shaking until the popping slows down, then immediately empty into the bowl.

4. Continue popping the amaranth in batches until you're all out of amaranth, or you've gotten too hungry to go on.

5. If you're using coconut oil, melt it in the pan and drizzle it over the amaranth. Other types of oil can be poured straight onto the amaranth. Season with salt and stir well. Enjoy immediately.

Nutrition: Calories: 83 Fat: 4g Carbohydrates: 10g Protein: 2g

34. Quickles

Preparation time: 5 minutes

Cooking time: 0 minutes

Servings: 4

Ingredients:

- 2 medium cucumbers or 1 large English cucumber (about 1 pound)
- 1½ tablespoons freshly squeezed lime juice
- ¼ teaspoon sea salt

Directions:

1. Wash the cucumber (no need to peel) and cut it into spears, about 2 inches long and ½-inch wide. Place in a bowl and toss with the lime juice and salt. Eat immediately.

Nutrition: Calories: 18 Fat: 0g Carbohydrates: 4g Protein: 3g

35. <u>Cinnamon Roll Energy Bites</u>

Preparation time: 15 minutes

Cooking time: 0 minutes

Servings: 18 bites

Ingredients:

- 1 cup walnuts
- 1 packed cup raisins
- 1 tablespoon ground cinnamon
- ¼ teaspoon sea salt
- ¼ teaspoon ground nutmeg

Directions:

1. In a food processor, combine the walnuts, raisins, cinnamon, salt, and nutmeg. Blend until the mixture balls up and sticks together.
2. With your hands, roll the mixture into 1-inch balls. Refrigerate in an airtight container for up to 2 months.

Nutrition: Calories: 71 Fat: 5g Carbohydrates: 8g Protein: 1g

36. Lemony Potato Veggie Bake

Preparation time: 10 minutes

Cooking time: 60 minutes

Servings: 6

Ingredients:

- 3½ cups finely diced potatoes (any variety, but red or gold are ideal)
- 1 (15-ounce) can chickpeas, drained &rinsed/1½ cups cooked chickpeas
- 1 medium red bell pepper, chopped
- ½ large white or yellow onion, chopped
- 1 cup broccoli florets
- ¼ cup freshly squeezed lemon juice
- 1 tablespoon olive oil
- 1 teaspoon sea salt
- ½ teaspoon freshly ground black pepper

Directions:

1. Preheat the oven to 400°F. Combine the potatoes, chickpeas, bell pepper, onion, broccoli, lemon juice, oil, salt, and pepper in a large bowl, and toss well to combine.

2. Transfer to two large nonstick baking sheets and spread into single layers. Bake for 30 minutes.

3. Toss and bake for another 20 to 30 minutes, or until the vegetables are browned and tender. Remove and enjoy.

Nutrition: Calories: 119 Fat: 2g Carbohydrates: 16g Protein: 2g

37. Edamame Miso Hummus

Preparation time: 15 minutes

Cooking time: 0 minutes

Servings: 6-8

Ingredients:

- 1¼ cups shelled edamame, thawed if frozen
- ½ cup tahini
- ½ cup baby spinach
- 5 tablespoons freshly squeezed lime juice
- 2 tablespoons water
- 1½ tablespoons mellow white miso
- 3 large garlic cloves, peeled
- ½ teaspoon sea salt

Directions:

1. In a blender, combine the edamame, tahini, spinach, lime juice, water, miso, garlic, and salt. Blend until completely smooth. Serve cold or at room temperature. Refrigerate in an airtight container for up to a week.

Nutrition: Calories: 131 Fat: 10g Carbohydrates: 6g Protein: 6g

38. Maple Shishitos

Preparation time: 5 minutes

Cooking time: 10 minutes

Servings: 4

Ingredients:

- Nonstick cooking spray (coconut oil)
- 1 pound shishito peppers, rinsed (no need to remove stems)
- 2 tablespoons maple syrup
- 4 teaspoons freshly squeezed lemon juice
- ¾ teaspoon sea salt

Directions:

1. Preheat the oven to broil. Spray a baking sheet with cooking spray. Put the peppers in a single layer on the baking sheet and spray the tops with oil.

2. Roast until the shishitos are browned with charred patches on them. This should take less than 10 minutes, so check on them every 2 minutes or so to prevent burning.

3. Remove from the oven. If they look dry, spritz with the oil again. Toss the peppers with the maple syrup,

lemon juice, and salt in a large bowl. Serve immediately.

Nutrition: Calories: 52 Fat: 0g Carbohydrates: 12g Protein: 3g

39. Garlic Mashed Potatoes

Preparation time: 5 minutes

Cooking time: 25 minutes

Servings: 4

Ingredients:

- 2 pounds russet or gold potatoes, peeled and chopped (6 cups)
- 1 cup water
- ½ cup raw unsalted whole cashews, soaked, drained, and rinsed
- 4 large garlic cloves, pressed or minced
- 1 teaspoon sea salt
- ½ teaspoon freshly ground black pepper

Directions:

1. Fill a large pot with some inches of water and bring to a boil. Place the potatoes in a steaming basket inside the pot. Cover and steam over medium heat for 25 minutes, or until fork tender.

2. Meanwhile, in a blender, combine the water and cashews. Blend until very smooth. Set aside. Drain or

strain the potatoes and transfer to a large bowl. Mash well with a potato masher or fork.

3. Add the cashew cream, garlic, salt, and pepper and whip with electric beaters, starting on low, then increasing to high, until very smooth and fluffy. Serve hot or warm.

Nutrition: Calories: 126 Fat: 3g Carbohydrates: 23g Protein: 4g

40. Ginger-Glazed Bok Choy

Preparation time: 5 minutes

Cooking time: 2 minutes

Servings: 3

Ingredients:

- 1 pound bok choy, chopped (about 16 cups)
- ¼ cup water
- 3 tablespoons minced fresh ginger
- 3 tablespoons tamari, shoyu, or soy sauce
- 1 tablespoon neutral-flavored oil (sunflower, sesame, or avocado)
- 2 tablespoons arrowroot powder

Directions:

1. Combine the bok choy, water, ginger, tamari, and oil in a large wok or skillet over medium-high heat.
2. Stir well, then sprinkle the arrowroot evenly over the top. Stir it in immediately. Cook within 2 minutes, stirring constantly, until the bok choy is wilted and crisp-tender. Serve immediately.

Nutrition: Calories: 74 Fat: 5g Carbohydrates: 6g Protein: 2g

DESSERT RECIPES

41. Banana Cream Pie

Preparation Time: 50 minutes

Cooking Time: 4 hours

Servings: 6

Ingredients:

- 1 1/2 cups dates, pitted and chopped
- 1 1/2 cups walnut
- 1/4 cup agave
- 1/4 teaspoon sea salt
- 6 ripe burro bananas, mashed
- 1 cup coconut milk, freshly squeezed
- 1 tablespoon chickpea flour
- 3/4 cup agave
- 1/8 teaspoon salt

Directions:

1. Prepare the pie crust. In a blender, mix the dates, walnuts, agave, and salt in a food processor. Pulse until

smooth. Press the pie crust into a pie pan. Place in the fridge then set aside to set.

2. Prepare the pie filling by placing the bananas, coconut milk, chickpea flour, agave, and salt in a food processor. Pulse until smooth. Place the filling into the prepared pie crust.

3. Place inside the Instant Pot. Close the lid but do not set the vent to the Sealing position. Press the Slow Cook button and adjust the cooking time to 4 hours.

Nutrition: Calories: 451 Protein: 6.5g Carbs: 63.9g; Fat: 23.2g

42. Spelt Raisin Balls

Preparation Time: 45 minutes

Cooking Time: 4 hours

Servings: 4

Ingredients:

- 1 and 1/2 cup spelt flour
- 1 and 1/2 cup dates, pitted and chopped
- 1/3 cup agave
- 1/3 cup grapeseed flour
- 1/2 teaspoon sea salt
- 1 cup seeded raisins, seeds removed and chopped

Directions:

1. Place all ingredients in a bowl. Mix until well-combined. Using your hands, form small balls and place each ball in the parchment-lined Instant Pot.

2. Close the lid but do not set the vent to the Sealing position. Press the Slow Cook button and adjust the cooking time to 4 hours. Make sure to flip the balls halfway through the cooking time.

Nutrition: Calories 428 Protein: 12gCarbs: 98.6gFat: 1.9g

43. <u>Applesauce</u>

Preparation Time: 20 minutes

Cooking Time: 20 minutes

Servings: 4

Ingredients:

- 3 cups peeled and cored apples, chopped
- 2 tablespoons agave
- 1 tablespoon lime juice, freshly squeezed
- 1/8 teaspoon cloves
- 1/8 teaspoon sea salt
- 1/2 cup strawberries
- 1 teaspoon sea moss
- 1/2 cup water

Directions:

1. Place all ingredients in a blender. Pulse until smooth. Pour mixture into the Instant Pot.

2. Press the Manual setting and adjust the cooking time to 10 minutes. Do natural pressure release to open the lid.

3. Once the lid is open, press the Sauté button and continue cooking until the applesauce thickens.

Nutrition: Calories: 64 Protein: 0.5g Carbs: 16.4gFat: 0.2g

44. Walnut Tahini Cups

Preparation Time: 55 minutes

Cooking Time: 4 hours

Servings: 4

Ingredients:

- 1 cup walnuts, pulsed using a food processor
- 1 tablespoon tahini
- 1/4 cup agave
- 2 tablespoons extra virgin coconut oil
- A pinch of sea salt

Directions:

1. Place all ingredients in a bowl. Mix until well-combined. Once the ingredients are well-combined, pour into silicone molds.
2. Place the molds inside the Instant Pot and close the lid. Do not set the vent to the Sealing position. Press the Slow Cook button and adjust the cooking time to 4 hours.

Nutrition: Calories: 228 Protein: 3.8g Carbs: 7g Fat: 21.9g

45. Chocolate Sea Salt Almonds

Preparation time: 40 minutes

Cooking time: 0 minutes

Servings: 8

Ingredients:

- 4 ounces low-carb chocolate, chopped
- 1 tablespoon coconut oil
- 1 cup dry-roasted almonds
- Sea salt

Directions:

1. Prepare a rimmed baking sheet lined using parchment paper. Dissolve the chocolate and coconut oil in a small saucepan over medium-low heat while stirring constantly.

2. Remove from the heat once melted and pour into a small bowl. Add the almonds to the chocolate and give them a good stir.

3. Using a teaspoon, remove a cluster of almonds and place it on the prepared baking sheet. Sprinkle with a bit of sea salt. Repeat this with the remaining nuts.

4. Put the baking sheet in the refrigerator within 30 minutes or until set. Remove and store the clusters in small resealable plastic bags in the refrigerator until ready to eat.

Nutrition: Calories: 187 Fat: 15g Protein: 6g Carbs: 7g

46. Salted Caramel Cashew Brittle

Preparation time: 1 hour & 10 minutes

Cooking time: 5 minutes

Servings: 6

Ingredients:

- 8 tablespoons grass-fed butter
- 4 tablespoons brown erythritol, granulated
- 4 ounces raw unsalted cashews
- 4 tablespoons natural cashew butter
- Coarse sea salt

Directions:

1. Prepare a rimmed baking sheet lined using parchment paper. In a small saucepan over low heat, stir the butter until it melts.

2. Add the erythritol, cashews, and cashew butter. Mix until thoroughly combined and melted. Pour the mixture onto the prepared baking sheet. Sprinkle salt on top.

3. Place the baking sheet in the refrigerator to harden for about 1 hour. Remove the brittle from the sheet and break into about 12 pieces.

4. Place each piece of brittle in a snack-size resealable plastic bag and store in the refrigerator or freezer for later use.

Nutrition: Calories: 321 Fat: 29g Protein: 5g Carbs: 10g

47. <u>Cookies and Cream Parfait</u>

Preparation time: 5 minutes

Cooking time: 0 minutes

Servings: 1

Ingredients:

- ½ scoop low-carb vanilla protein powder
- ¾ cup plain full-fat Greek yogurt
- 1 Oreo cookie
- 4 tablespoons sugar-free chocolate syrup

Directions:

1. Mix the protein powder and Greek yogurt in a small bowl until smooth and creamy. Remove one side of the Oreo cookie.

2. Place it in a small resealable plastic bag and crush it with the back of a spoon. Set aside. Pour the chocolate syrup over the yogurt mixture and sprinkle with the cookie crumbles.

Nutrition: Calories: 281 Fat: 13g Protein: 19g Carbs: 22g

48. Pecan Pie Pudding

Preparation time: 5 minutes

Cooking time: 0 minutes

Servings: 1

Ingredients:

- ¾ cup plain full-fat Greek yogurt
- ½ scoop low-carb vanilla protein powder
- 4 tablespoons chopped pecans
- 2 tablespoons sugar-free syrup

Directions:

1. Mix the Greek yogurt plus protein powder in a small bowl until smooth and creamy. Top with the chopped pecans and syrup.

Nutrition: Calories: 381 Fat: 21g Protein: 32g Carbs: 16g

49. <u>Chocolate Avocado Pudding</u>

Preparation time: 5 minutes

Cooking time: 0 minutes

Servings: 1

Ingredients:

- 1 avocado, halved
- 1/3 cup full-fat coconut milk
- 1 teaspoon vanilla extract
- 2 tablespoons unsweetened cocoa powder
- 5 or 6 drops liquid stevia

Directions:

1. Combine all the fixings in a high-powered blender or food processor and blend until smooth. Serve immediately.

Nutbition: Calories: 555 Fat: 47g Protein: 7g Carbs: 26g

50. "Frosty" Chocolate Shake

Preparation time: 40 minutes

Cooking time: 0 minutes

Servings: 2

Ingredients:

- 1 cup heavy (whipping) cream/coconut cream
- 2 tablespoons unsweetened cocoa powder
- 1 tablespoon almond butter
- 1 teaspoon vanilla extract
- 5 or 6 drops liquid stevia

Directions:

1. Beat the cream in a medium bowl or using a stand mixer until fluffy, 3 to 4 minutes. Add the cocoa powder, almond butter, vanilla, and stevia.

2. Beat the mixture for an additional 2 to 3 minutes, or until the mixture has the consistency of whipped cream. Place the bowl in the freezer for 25 to 30 minutes before serving.

Nutrition: Calories: 493 Fat: 49g Protein: 5g Carbs: 8g

CONCLUSION

Following a plant based diet is an amazing way to maintain a healthy lifestyle and to stay fit. By eating a diet very rich in fruits, vegetables, and whole grains, you'll be protecting your body from developing heart disease, diabetes, and cancer, just to name a few. Plant-based diets may be considered to be healthy because they eliminate or drastically limit meat, dairy, and eggs, which are associated with increased risks of cardiovascular disease, high blood pressure, obesity, and diabetes. the plant based diet is a diet that focuses on consuming foods that are derived from plants, rather than from animals. There are various types of plant-based diets, all of which emphasise different combinations of foods.

Grains are essential of plant based diet and can be found in the seeds of a number of different grasses. Wheat, oats, rice, cornmeal, and barley are among the many varieties available. When grains are first harvested, they are considered whole, with their most essential components intact: bran and germ. These grains are stripped of their bran and germ, as well as their essential nutrients, during processing. This produces processed and enriched grains, which are used to make products like white bread and white rice, which have a longer shelf life. As you probably already know, these foods are not really good. Look for the terms processed or enriched grains on food labels and avoid them. The nutrients lost in processed grains are never substituted. The goods in enriched grains are fortified with the nutrients that have been stripped out, but they do not give the same benefits as consuming whole foods with the natural nutrients from the start.

CPSIA information can be obtained
at www.ICGtesting.com
Printed in the USA
BVHW091148150621
609530BV00013B/2631